Birth Control

for CHRISTIANS

Birth Control *for* CHRISTIANS

D. B. RYEN

© 2020 D. B. Ryen Incorporated

Version 1.3

All rights reserved.

No part of this book may be reproduced or transmitted for the purpose of profit or monetary gain in any form or by any means, electronic or physical, including photocopying, recording, or any information storage and retrieval system – except by a reviewer who may quote brief passages in a review to be printed in a magazine, newspaper, or on the internet – without permission in writing from the publisher and/or author. However, replication and/or distribution free of charge is acceptable.

Although the author has made every effort to ensure the accuracy and completeness of the information contained in this book, we assume no responsibility for errors, inaccuracies, omissions, or any inconsistency herein.

All instances of biblical quotes are either original translations, loosely paraphrased from various biblical sources, or used with permission from *THE STORY OF JESUS: ALL FOUR GOSPELS IN ONE*.

Contact us at: email@dbryen.com

Visit our website at: www.dbryen.com

ISBN: 9798642050088

Cover photo: public domain

Table of Contents

PREFACE
    The Backstory   9

PART 1: THE SCIENCE
    Introduction   15
    Girl Parts   16
    Guy Parts   19
    Baby Parts   20

PART 2: THE ETHICS
    The Big Issue   29
    Two Required Steps   31
    When Personhood Begins   31
    To Use or Not To Use   39
    A Sensitive Topic   41
    Summary   43

PART 3: THE METHODS
    Introduction   47
    Conservative   48

Barrier	52
Hormones	54
Long Term	59
Permanent	64
Breastfeeding	66
Emergency Contraception	67
Abstinence	69

PART 4: REPRODUCTIVE TECHNOLOGY

Introduction	73
Options	74
Summary	78

CONCLUSION

Final Words	81

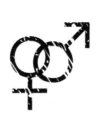

Preface

The Backstory

Shortly after college, I got a desk job. One day a co-worker walked into my office and sat down. She asked me whether I knew anything about birth control.

"Uh... what do you mean?"

She was getting married in a month and didn't want to get pregnant for a couple years, but she was nervous about what kind of birth control to use.

"Aren't there some kinds that, like, cause an abortion every month? I don't want anything like that. I want something that doesn't even let the sperm meet the egg."

She knew I'd studied Natural Sciences with a thesis on the ethics of cloning. Cloning technology deals with embryos, which many feel are simply little people waiting to grow up. The ethics of cloning has to do with the beginning of *personhood*, that is, when a new human life begins. This same issue also applies to the ethics of birth control. If a couple feels that life begins at fertilization (when the sperm and egg combine), they may not like the idea of contraception that potentially allows that to happen.

The science of birth control can be baffling to anyone without a medical degree, and the ethics can be overwhelming to anyone without a philosophy degree. It seems like everyone has a different opinion on what methods are right or wrong, and condemnation of other views is rampant. Misinformation is prevalent, further contributing to misunderstanding. It's no wonder my colleague needed some guidance.

She's not alone.

Like many women, she didn't fully understand what happened inside her every month during her cycle. Most men are clueless. And since there are so many different birth control products on the market, each working to prevent pregnancy in a different way, choosing one can be daunting.

Anytime people run up against a controversial topic – a moral gray zone – I find it best to simply present all the available information and let each person make an informed decision for themselves. That's what this book is all about: education. We'll look at the science behind birth control and explore some of the major moral viewpoints. However, I'll stop short of recommending a particular method – that's between each couple and God, based on their individual convictions and beliefs. Whatever your situation, there's a good method of birth control for you and your spouse (or future spouse). Rest assured that none of the methods in this book cause an abortion, that is, they don't harm an existing pregnancy.

This book is geared toward women, since the majority of birth control methods involves their reproductive system, but men should also read this book in its entirety. Birth control and the ethics surrounding reproduction involve both of you. It takes two to tango. If nothing else, most men would benefit from a better understanding of their partner's monthly cycle, which is something that each couple must manage together. After all, your body belongs to the other,[1] and should be lovingly cared for accordingly.

Disclaimer: this book does not replace the advice of your doctor. *Birth Control For Christians* can help you learn some of the facts surrounding reproduction, and some of the different ethical issues, but it's not meant to be your only resource. Discuss your birth control goals with your doctor in the privacy and confidentiality of a quiet exam room. Nothing should replace the advice of a licenced physician you trust and respect.

Throughout this book, I encourage you to have an open mind. Share your thoughts with your partner and try to keep the whole thing lighthearted. Birth control is a serious topic, with implications for everything from reproductive technology to pregnancy terminations to the possibility of human cloning. But, most of all, it's a topic that pertains to a particularly enjoyable act in the context of a loving, committed relationship. Being overly solemn won't help matters. Whatever you and your partner choose should be well-understood, easy to use, and (most of all) keep your conscience clear.

So, without further delay, let's get into it.

Enjoy!

---

[1] 1 Corinthians 7:4

Part 1: The Science

Introduction

Before we talk about how the various methods of birth control work, we need to understand the basic science of reproduction.

Birth control works in one of three ways: (1) interfering with the menstrual cycle, (2) blocking sperm from getting into the uterus, or (3) preventing implantation of an embryo in the uterus. That's it. So, to understand how each method works, we first need to understand: (1) how the normal menstrual cycle works, (2) how sperm get into the uterus (I'm sure you've already figured this one out), and (3) how babies form in the womb.

Making an informed decision about birth control requires a basic understanding of how reproduction works. This can be daunting, but bear with me. We'll try to make things simple, and keep medical jargon to a minimum. We'll only discuss the *relevant* points, and, hopefully, by the end you'll feel much more comfortable with the complex biologic processes that happen inside us every day.

If the science of reproduction doesn't interest you, and you just want to know your birth control options, feel free to skip ahead. After all, this is a book – you can flip back here for clarification anytime.

That being said, let's dive in to the most intimidating subject of all: the menstrual cycle.

Girl Parts

The menstrual cycle is the natural series of changes that occur every month in women. There are hormones, ovulation, premenstrual symptoms (PMS), and periods (bleeding).

In terms of hormones, the only ones you need to know about are estrogen and progesterone. In the first half of the cycle, estrogen goes up. In the second half of the cycle, progesterone goes up. The lining of the uterus changes monthly in response to these fluctuating hormones. When they both taper off, a period happens.

DAY 1-13

Your cycle starts on the first day of your period. Your brain tells your ovaries to start making eggs. Not just one egg. Lots of eggs. But although many eggs start developing, just one gets released. The egg with the best development becomes dominant while all the others stop growing at various stages and fade away.

Each developing egg and the cells surrounding it are collectively called a *follicle*. Developing follicles produce estrogen and release it into the bloodstream. Estrogen triggers the lining of the uterus to get thicker. So, at the same time as the egg is developing, the lining of the uterus is getting ready for its release.

Follow me so far? An egg develops in the ovaries while the uterine lining gets thicker. Estrogen goes up. That's the first part of the cycle.

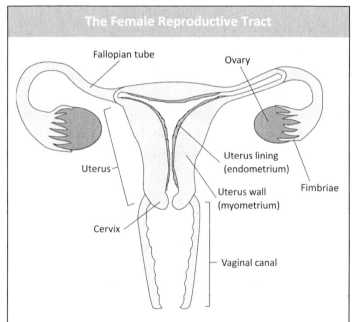

Figure 1: Look familiar? It's what's inside each woman. And it's complicated. Does anyone without a medical degree actually understand how all of it works? That's what we'll soon learn all about.

Ovaries are about the size and shape of big grapes. The uterus is like an upside-down pear, but expands to the size of a watermelon during pregnancy.

Day 14

Next comes ovulation. In a 28-day cycle, ovulation occurs on Day 14. As the dominant follicle matures, the brain releases a surge of hormones that causes the follicle to burst open and the egg to be released from the ovary.

Some women feel mild pain during ovulation, typically on one side of their abdomen. Sometimes there's spotting. Many women don't notice ovulation at all. Either way, ovulation's a big deal: it's essential to fertility, and it signals the transition into the second part of the menstrual cycle.

Day 15-28

The *fimbriae* of the fallopian tubes are waiting for the newly-released egg. They gently sweep it down toward the uterus. The whole journey down the tube takes the better part of a week. It's during this time the egg may or may not meet one lucky sperm and become fertilized. Let's just assume there are no sperm in this cycle and the egg continues on unfertilized. We'll talk more about fertilization and pregnancy later.

Although the big follicle in the ovary has released its egg, its job isn't done. The follicle now starts producing progesterone, the second important hormone in the menstrual cycle. Progesterone stabilizes the uterine lining so it stays thick, but not so thick that it starts falling apart. The uterine lining – after two weeks of estrogen and about a week of progesterone – is just right for a fertilized egg to implant and cause a pregnancy.

However, in most menstrual cycles, nothing implants in the uterine lining. Without implantation, the ovary runs out of steam: the empty follicle stops producing progesterone and the uterine lining starts falling apart. This is the time women get *premenstrual syndrome* (PMS), which is any sort of unpleasant symptom that signals your period is coming soon. Cramping, irritability, increased appetite, sadness, fatigue, and breast tenderness are some of the most common PMS symptoms.

DAY 1-7

Without a pregnancy, the uterine lining sheds itself. This causes bleeding and cramping. The thickness that was built up during the previous cycle gets sloughed off and empties out the cervix into the vaginal canal.

Then the whole cycle starts again. The ovaries heal up and start producing a fresh batch of follicles. After menstruation (a period), the uterine lining starts building up again from the estrogen released by the follicles.

NORMAL'S NOT ALWAYS NORMAL

All that describes a normal menstrual cycle. However, as most women will tell you, abnormal cycles are common. All sorts of things can go awry with the brain's hormones, follicle development, estrogen and progesterone, the uterine lining, bleeding, and any other aspect of the menstrual cycle. We won't get into any of them here. If you have abnormalities with your cycle, talk to your doctor; often there are treatments available for various problematic conditions.

Guy Parts

Okay, we've tackled the female reproductive system. Not too bad? The next reproductive system is much less complicated. In fact, it's downright simple. We don't need to discuss any anatomy or hormones – all you need to know is that men produced sperm. Lots and lots of sperm. Millions are released during intercourse,

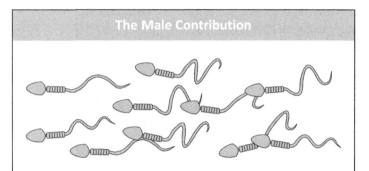

Figure 2: Yep, those are the man's swimmers. Sperm. Don't they look so happy to be swimming free? The race is on.

but only one can fertilize an egg.

Sperm are produced in the testicles, but semen is the product of a number of different glands in the male reproductive system. After intercourse, the sperm go to work. Their job is to swim into the cervix (the opening of the uterus), through the uterus, find a fallopian tube, and fertilize the egg.

Once a single sperm binds to an egg, a new cell is created with new DNA. This is the first step in producing new life.

Baby Parts

Now that we've covered the female and male reproductive systems, we turn to what happens when they come together to make a new person. This is fetal development, or, in everyday language, how babies are made.

First, let's define a few words so we're all on the same page. An *embryo* is the early stages of development of a new baby. Whether it's one cell or many cells, it's called an embryo until about eight weeks after fertilization. At this point, all of the major organ systems have formed, although they're not fully functional until later on. From the ninth week onward, the new life is called a *fetus*. Only after birth does this new life officially become a baby. Not before. Although most people use these terms interchangeably (even doctors will refer to the "baby" growing inside you), we'll try stick with the official definitions in this book to avoid confusion. This whole topic is confusing enough as it is.

FERTILIZATION

The first biological step in the development of a new person is fertilization. As we discussed, a sperm swims through the uterus and fallopian tube to look for an egg.

The most fertile time in the menstrual cycle is the two days leading up to ovulation. So if ovulation occurs around Day 14 of the menstrual cycle, a woman is most likely to get pregnant with intercourse during Days 12-14.

If the timing is ideal, the sperm will meet the egg just after it bursts out of the ovary. The first sperm to successfully fuse with the egg triggers a chemical reaction that prevents other sperm from binding. Within the egg, the half-set of DNA from the father combines with the half-set of DNA from the mother to produce a full set of new DNA. That's fertilization: a sperm plus an egg equals a new cell.

At this point, the new cell is called a *zygote*. This is the first stage in embryonic development. The zygote is a single cell with a complete set of DNA, and it begins replicating right away. The single cell divides to become two, then four, then eight, and so on. Each has its own copy of DNA. Within a few days, there's a cluster of cells, each a replica of the original. At this point, the embryo is called a *morula*. All the cells in the morula are the same; none of them have differentiated into other cell types. They each have the potential to become any type of specialized cell within the new body.

I'm sure you're already a bit overwhelmed with all the stages the embryo goes through. But these early steps are important, as we'll see later.

During those first few days after fertilization, as the new cells are replicating, the embryo drifts down the fallopian tube and arrives in the main part of the uterus. By this time, the cells that were all the same have started to *differentiate*, that is, they become different from one another. Some cells form an outer layer, some cells form an inner layer. A pocket of fluid develops within the outer layer, pushing the inner cells to one side. Now that we have different cell types, the morula has matured into a *blastocyst*. This is the stage that implantation occurs at.

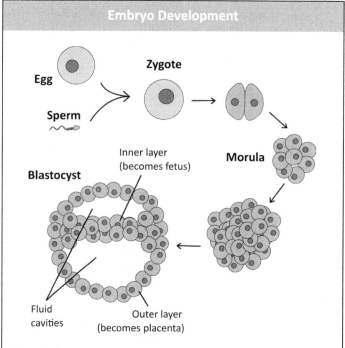

Figure 3: These steps are the basics of early embryology. The names don't matter as much as the progression of complexity, particularly around the time of implantation.

Lost yet? Look at the diagram to get an overview of what we've just discussed. To summarize:
1. Sperm combines with egg (fertilization)
2. One cell (zygote) becomes cluster of cells (morula)
3. Cluster of cells migrates down to uterus
4. Cells form different layers (blastocyst)

So now we have an embryo floating in the uterus, ready to implant. This next step is critical.

IMPLANTATION

Around Day 21, the lining of the uterus is ready to receive the embryo. Implantation is when the embryo (at the blastocyst stage) gets stuck to the lining of the uterus. Uterus cells wrap around the embryo, and the embryo burrows into the lining of the uterus. Implantation is usually complete 8-10 days after fertilization, or around Day 23 of the menstrual cycle.

Then a whole bunch of stuff happens at once. Because their cells are now touching, the mother and embryo start passing chemical signals to each other. This communication makes both the uterus and embryo shift gears and start developing like crazy.

Let's start with the embryo. Although some differentiation has already occurred to get to the blastocyst stage, the embryo's cells start differentiating even more and adopting different roles. Cell layers fold and loop on themselves, forming tubes and discs and more pockets of fluid. The embryo develops different ends, which become the head and backside of the fetus.

The uterus starts changing too. Up until this point, the embryo as been receiving nutrients from the fluid inside the uterus. But as the embryo grows, a greater supply is needed. Thus, a placenta develops. Uterine cells around the embryo develop extra blood vessels to feed nutrients to the newly-implanted embryo. Hormones from the placenta tell the brain and ovaries to maintain progesterone production and prevent menstruation.

All in all, an embryo progresses from a cluster of cells casually travelling down the fallopian tube to complex arrangement of cell layers embedded within the uterine lining that communicates via chemicals to its mother and starts forming a placenta. As you can see, a lot happens after implantation, and it all happens in a matter of days. But the big picture is that this flurry of activity has triggered changes in the woman that we call *pregnancy*.

Now, just a note about *conception*. This a confusing term. It can refer to fertilization or implantation, depending who you ask. It can also imply that a new person has formed. We'll avoid using the word "conception" altogether, since it can be a source of misunderstanding.

Fetal Development

A note about twins: sometimes multiple eggs are released from the ovaries during ovulation. These individual eggs each have the potential to become fertilized and implant in the uterus. That's how fraternal (*non-identical*) twins are produced. Or triplets. Or quadruplets. They all have their own placentas.

However, *identical* twins occur when a single embryo splits into two. Because the cells are all identical, both clusters develop into identical fetuses. They may or may not share a placenta.

Regardless of how many embryos implant, a fully mature fetus develops within the next 38 weeks, with organs that are completely functional and ready to maintain life independent of its mother. Any defects or deviations in development can be catastrophic, leading to pregnancy loss or congenital abnormalities with a wide range of outcomes. We won't get into those here – we'll just assume normal fetal development for the purposes of our discussion.

Sometime later in the pregnancy, the fetus comes out of the uterus. This occurs either via vaginal delivery or C-section. Either way, the *fetus* becomes a *baby* as it leaves the uterus. The placenta is no longer needed and is discarded after birth.

The Bottom Line

The tricky part, ethically, is this: when exactly does a collection of cells become a new person? It may seem arbitrary, but your answer may determine what type of birth control you'll be comfortable using. It also has implications for reproductive technology, stem cell research, and pregnancy termination. For many couples, when personhood begins is a big deal.

That's what the next section is all about.

Part 2: The Ethics

The Big Issue

We're swimming in the deep end now. Gone is the shallow end of the pool, where our feet can firmly touch bottom. There's no question of what happens *biologically* during the development of an embryo, but there are many questions about what happens *philosophically* during that same period.

There's been a lot of moral controversy surrounding various topics in reproduction. These include methods of contraception (birth control), abortion, in vitro fertilization, and stem cell research, among others. We'll get to all those individually, but they all essentially boil down to one common denominator. This is the issue of personhood. As we've said, the big question is this:

when has a new person begun? That's what this next section hinges on.

Personhood means the essence of what it means to be human, not just possessing a physical body but having a soul. It's the non-physical stuff of our being, however you define that.

We'll explore various answers to when personhood begins by examining the Bible, logic, historical perspectives, and various common viewpoints. However, throughout this discussion, keep in mind that nobody knows for sure when a person begins. Everyone has an opinion about it, but God alone knows the truth. As humans, we try to grasp God's truth, but ultimately fail to comprehend it completely because we don't have his perspective.[1] And yet, we *should* strive to pursue God's ultimate truth, even if it's not possible for us to fully understand.

Every couple must draw their own line in the sand, so to speak. That is, you have to decide with your partner when you think personhood begins, based on sound information and reasoning.

As with the prior section, if this issue isn't a big deal to you, move on. Skip to the third section of this book and pick a method of birth control that is the most convenient for you. No problem. Breathe easy and use birth control with a clear conscience.

However, if this issue *is* a big deal to you, consider all of the perspectives discussed here, pick the one that you feel best represents your understanding, and act accordingly. Nobody can make the decision for you, nor can anyone tell you it's wrong. This is between you and your partner. And God. Do your best, then walk forward guilt-free. As the Bible says, *"It was for freedom that Christ set us free,"*[2] and *"the one who examines me is the Lord,"*[3] not other people.

---

[1] Isaiah 55:8-9; Isaiah 40:13-14

[2] Galatians 5:1

[3] 1 Corinthians 4:4

Two Required Steps

Two things are absolutely required to make a baby: fertilization and implantation. One without the other won't allow for reproduction. Ever. Both are absolutely essential.

Probably.[1]

First, fertilization is a requirement for reproduction. A sperm fertilizes an egg, new DNA is created, and new life begins to grow.

Second, implantation is a requirement for reproduction. An embryo must implant in a uterus for development to progress beyond the earliest stages. Contrary to what you've seen in the movies, a baby can never be grown in a lab. Fertilization may occur outside a womb, but in order to progress beyond the blastocyst stage, an embryo must implant. Babies being grown in a lab is completely fictional. A functional placenta, which only develops after implantation, is an absolute requirement for reproduction.

When Personhood Begins

There's a whole spectrum of beliefs about when personhood begins. We won't go into all of them here, but we'll explore some of the most common ones. As we said before, none are right or wrong. All make sense on some level, and all have challenges.

---

[1] We'll see later how fertilization can *theoretically* be bypassed, and that implantation elsewhere in the body (outside the uterus) can very rarely produce a live birth.

AT BIRTH

Genesis states that *"the LORD God formed man from the dust of the ground and breathed into his nose the breath of life, and man became a living soul."*[1] So does personhood begin at birth, when a baby takes its first breath?

This is the current basis of criminal law. A fetus doesn't hold the rights of a baby. Assault of a pregnant woman, even if it equally harms her fetus, is still considered a crime against one person, not two. There's some consideration for a fetus becoming injured before birth *if* it proceeds to be born alive. But if the fetus dies before birth (i.e. a miscarriage), it has no rights. The fetus must be completely independent of its mother to be considered a baby — the umbilical cord must be cut, the lungs must be full of air.

This definition of personhood doesn't seem right to many people. Why should a fetus not hold the rights of a baby breathing on its own? The two states may be only moments apart. Does the soul enter the body only when the first breath is taken?

Many would argue it happens long before.

Mothers often claim they knew the personality of their baby well before they were born: strong-willed or easy-going, restless or content. The characteristics we see in adults are often present at birth, and even before birth.

The Bible also suggests personhood begins before birth.

"The LORD called me from the womb, and from my mother's belly he named me."[2]

"Before I formed you in the womb, I knew you. Before you came out of the womb, I consecrated you."[3]

"He'll be filled with the Holy Spirit from his mother's womb."[4]

---

[1] Genesis 2:7

[2] Isaiah 49:1

[3] Jeremiah 1:5

[4] Luke 1:15

> "When Elizabeth heard Mary's greeting, the baby leaped in her womb."[1]
>
> "When God, who consecrated me from my mother's womb and called me by his grace..."[2]

It's clear that God knew us before we were born, which suggests we had a soul and a personality that could be known.

Let's re-examine Genesis 2:7. Can becoming *"a living soul"* occur before the process of breathing *"into his nose the breath of life"*? After all, the way Adam was formed from the dust is quite a bit different from how the rest of us were formed in the womb.

Personhood beginning before birth is suggested both by the Bible and basic reasoning. This viewpoint is not fact, but it's intuitive. Regardless of what the law states, it seems like our souls are with us well before we're born.

However, exactly when we become *"living souls"* is open to debate.

FERTILIZATION

Undoubtedly, biological life begins at fertilization. The sperm and egg unite to form a new set of genetic material (DNA). Immediately, the zygote begins replicating independent of its parents. This is one of the most popular milestones for when personhood begins, and for good reason: the embryo is a brand-new creature, at least physically.

One of the challenges with personhood beginning at fertilization is the vast number of fertilized eggs that fail to implant. There's no way to know the exact number, but for sexually active couples not using birth control, an egg likely gets fertilized during most (if not all) menstrual cycles. However, due to any number of

---

[1] Luke 1:41
[2] Galatians 1:15

issues, the embryo doesn't always implant in the uterine lining. Most commonly, the timing of fertilization was too late – if fertilization occurs a number of days *after* ovulation, the embryo isn't ready for implantation by the time it reaches the uterus. In this case, the new "person" would be flushed out of the uterus with the woman's next period. Arguably, more fertilized eggs fail to implant than actually cause pregnancies. So, if personhood begins at fertilization, the majority of "people" would never make it past existing as a tiny cluster of cells (morula) before being expelled from the uterus and dying.

This seems illogical. Why would God create the majority of people just to live a few days as a featureless collection of cells? Do they all go to heaven? Hell? Are they even people at all?

Another challenge is that of identical twins, which arise from a division of a single embryo. Their DNA is the same. After they split, they develop independently of each other. But if personhood begins at fertilization, are there two souls within that single first cell (zygote)? Or do they become individual people upon splitting? Or is the embryo a single person until the split, and then the second embryo becomes a person as well?

There are no definitive answers to these existential questions. But they pose a logical challenge to the idea that personhood begins at fertilization.

IMPLANTATION

Implantation is the second critical step in the development of a new baby. If implantation doesn't occur, the embryo doesn't move past the blastocyst stage. Ever. So is implantation when an embryo becomes a person?

Perhaps. Consider the most famous prenatal passage in the Bible:

> *"For you created my organs; you wove me together in my mother's womb.*
> *I thank you because I'm fearfully and uniquely made....*
> *My bones weren't hidden from you when I was made in secret, when I was woven together in the depths of the earth.*
> *Your eyes saw me forming."*[1]

Now, let's go out on a limb – bear with me as we explore this passage. David talks about "parts" being woven together. This implies that there are different parts in the developing body. An embryo at the morula stage is just a cluster of cells, all of which are the same. No "parts," just one "part." An embryo at the blastocyst stage has different layers of cells, thus it has "parts" that can be woven together. This is right around the time of implantation. So maybe the Bible suggests that personhood *doesn't* begin at fertilization, when there is no cellular differentiation; rather, it's at or after implantation, when the embryo has different parts.

Perhaps, but the logic here is a stretch.

It's highly unlikely King David had extensive knowledge of early fetal development when he wrote Psalm 139. The Psalms aren't science textbooks, they're poetry. So to use this passage to imply personhood begins at a certain time is probably an inappropriate interpretation. Still, if the Bible suggests a time that an unborn baby becomes a person, it's at or after implantation, not just at fertilization. The cellular differentiation and interaction with the mother are key.

However, there are logical challenges with this view too.

What about pregnancies that don't have a chance at surviving until birth? A normal human cell has 46 chromosomes, 23 from each parent. The majority of first trimester miscarriages occur because of major chromosomal abnormalities. That is, the sperm or the egg contributes an extra chromosome to the genetic profile,

---
[1] Psalm 139:13-16

or is missing a full chromosome, or has an extra half-set of chromosomes. These major genetic abnormalities aren't compatible with life.

What about those pregnancies? Were those people too? They had unique DNA (albeit abnormal), and the embryo successfully implanted and started developing further, but there was no chance of survival till birth.

There's also the case of ectopic pregnancies. This is when an embryo implants itself somewhere other than the inside of the uterus. It can be in a fallopian tube (most common), the cervix, fimbriae, an ovary, or elsewhere in the abdomen (rare). Only a uterus can support a growing fetus, and implantation anywhere else will not survive until birth.[1] Indeed, the mother's life is in danger if she doesn't receive urgent medical attention to terminate the pregnancy.

Does the fetus of an ectopic pregnancy have a soul? It has gone through fertilization and has new DNA. It has implanted (albeit in the wrong place) and started developing further beyond the blastocyst state. An early placenta forms. Is the fetus of an ectopic pregnancy a person?

In all of these cases – abnormal DNA and abnormal implantation – the fetus doesn't even have a chance at life outside the womb. So should we consider them people?

There's no good answer to this. God alone knows.

DURING PREGNANCY

As we've seen, according to the Bible and basic logic, it's reasonable to conclude that personhood begins before birth. Many people feel this way. However, if personhood doesn't begin at the

---

[1] Abdominal pregnancies occur when implantation occurs in the abdomen, away from the uterus, fallopian tubes, and ovaries. This is a very rare type of ectopic pregnancy. It's extremely unlikely the baby will survive.

moment of fertilization or implantation, there are various other milestones during pregnancy that could be considered the beginning of personhood.

However, before we get into that, we should talk about fetal age. Embryonic and gestational age aren't the same thing. Embryonic (or fetal) age refers to the age of the developing baby from the moment of fertilization. That's Day 1. Gestational age, however, starts counting the age of a fetus based on the mother's menstrual cycle. Day 1 is the same Day 1 of your cycle – the first day of your period. In a typical cycle, fertilization occurs on Day 14. Even though the embryo is actually brand new (embryonic age Day 1), the gestational age is 14 days. Embryonic age and gestational age are two weeks apart. Likewise, implantation occurs around Week 1 embryonically, but Week 3 gestationally. Doctors predominantly use gestational age to talk about pregnancy. Your estimated due date is 40 weeks after the first day of your last period, which corresponds to an embryonic age of 38 weeks.

When we're discussing early fetal development in this book, we use embryonic age (starts with fertilization) when referring to the first few weeks after the sperm and egg come together. But in the odd instance we discuss full term babies, or anything out of the first trimester, we'll use gestational age (starts at your period). We'll try to clarify if there's any confusion, like in this instance where we list milestones in embryonic age early on, but switch to gestational age when the baby becomes viable outside the womb (around 24 weeks gestational age, 22 weeks embryonic age).

This can be terribly confusing for the general public. So, on behalf of the entire worldwide medical community, I apologize.

Now, back to when personhood begins. Here are some of the major developmental milestones during pregnancy:

- Week 3: heart begins to beat
- Week 6: organized brain activity

- Week 9: movements (not purposeful); major organ systems formed; embryo now called a fetus
- Week 12: swallowing; movements (purposeful)
- Week 24: viability (the baby can survive with full medical care if born this early)
- Week 37: considered full term
- Week 40: official due date

Any given milestone, or more, could be considered the beginning of personhood. The Bible suggests that personhood begins before birth, but it doesn't say exactly when a developing baby gets a soul.

Take your pick. Again, your informed choice is as good as any.

After Birth

In contrast to personhood beginning well *before* birth, early societies didn't consider babies to be people until *well after* birth. This was primarily because of high infant mortality. Even up until the 1900s, about a third of babies didn't survive until their second birthday. Infection was the primary cause of early childhood death; accidental deaths (falls, fire, drowning) were common too. Abandonment – because of gender, twin pregnancies, or birth defects – has led to the deaths of many newborns even into the 20th century. As a result, many cultures throughout history didn't consider newborn babies as people. It was just too common for babies to die before they'd learned to walk that they didn't receive the same consideration as older children. Indeed, the practice of recording the age of children is relatively new.

This idea may seem barbaric to us now, but our ancestors likely had far different ideas of personhood than we do currently. Quite frankly, it was a different world back then.

PICK YOUR PLACE

You and your partner have to draw your line in the sand somewhere, wherever your conscience is comfortable. Make an informed decision, then do your best to not let judgment or condemnation from others affect your decision. It's between you, your partner, and God.

To Use or Not To Use

We mentioned earlier that the whole issue of reproductive ethics hinges on our view of when personhood begins. However, regardless of that perspective, every couple must first decide *if* they want to use birth control at all. Now, if you're reading this book, you and your partner have probably decided you want birth control of some sort. However, it's worth considering whether birth control itself fits with your belief system.

God said, *"Be fruitful and multiply."*[1] Some would view birth control as a deliberate violation of that early command. Various church denominations adhere to this view. They consider each pregnancy a blessing and each child a reward. Why actively prevent something that God designed to be a good thing?

The official stance of the Roman Catholic church is against birth control in general. Their argument is both thoughtful and biblical. Essentially, married love should always be open to new life, which is often the case within a marriage. For instance, when a husband and wife get pregnant, even if they are actively trying *not* to, what's their reaction? It's typically positive. "Oh well, I guess we're having a baby." A pregnancy may cause lots of added stress, but most will figure out a way to make it work. Married

---

[1] Genesis 1:28

couples in a healthy relationship will typically welcome a child, even if its arrival was unplanned.

On the other hand, when an unmarried couple gets pregnant, what's the reaction? Often fear, anxiety, and regret. "Oh no, this is awful. What am I going to do?" Notice that the difficulty is more often faced individually when unmarried ("What am *I* going to do?") rather than together as a married couple ("What are *we* going to do?"). The commitment that comes with a marriage changes the dynamic of parenthood completely. If the parents are unmarried, the baby may still be raised in a loving home, but the social situation is more precarious. The likelihood of terminating the pregnancy is higher.

There's also an argument that birth control leads to promiscuity. It's difficult to definitively prove whether sexual sin has increased since the introduction of birth control, but it's not an unreasonable claim. However, regardless of the prevalence of promiscuity and "free love," the use of birth control doesn't necessarily mean individual people are more or less likely to have sex outside marriage. Especially within the context of a marriage, using birth control is a reasonable consideration for most couples. Intercourse outside of marriage and birth control are different moral issues – it's a false assumption to state that one will lead to the other. There's no question that the two issues are related, but the cause-and-effect argument is a slippery slope.

That said, if you're reading this, you're probably already set on using birth control. There are many other books that can address the issue of sexual sin far better than this one.

So let's move on.

A Sensitive Topic

In medical school, I worked with an obstetrician who had done extra training in maternal-fetal medicine, which specializes in problems during pregnancy. Quite out of the blue, while waiting for a C-section to start, he asked me, "How do you feel about abortions?"

A controversial topic, to say the least.

Before we go further, let's clarify some terminology again. An *abortion* is the end of a fetus' life before birth. If it's unintentional and occurs before 20 weeks gestation, doctors call that a *spontaneous* abortion. After 20 weeks, unintentional fetal loss is called a *miscarriage*. However, if the pregnancy is deliberately terminated at any time, it's called a *therapeutic* abortion. This is a misnomer, since there's typically nothing therapeutic about it. For our purposes here, we'll call any intentional pregnancy termination an abortion and any unintentional pregnancy loss a miscarriage, in keeping with how the general public uses those terms.

Despite the negative stigma, pregnancy termination is one of the most frequently performed surgeries in the developed world. However, the medical community as a whole (at least where I trained) doesn't discriminate anymore against doctors who support or oppose abortion. There's a general understanding that abortion is a personal decision. Some doctors are okay with it, some aren't, but most of them respect the right of everyone to choose for themselves. Nobody – not even trainees, like I was at the time – was expected to participate in performing an abortion if they didn't want to. No pressure, no questions asked.

So, when my staff physician asked me about my views, I felt it nonjudgmentally.

"I'm not really okay with it," I replied. "I get that it still happens and we have a duty to care for our patients regardless of our views, but I don't think I could be a part of that process for any of my patients."

"Yes, yes," he said. "I feel the same. I'm Catholic. But it's a different story, you know, when it's *you* in that position."

He went on to explain that he's had many patients who were adamantly opposed to abortion but found themselves in the position of having an unexpected and/or unwanted pregnancy. Sometimes it was due to a genetic or developmental problem with the fetus. Sometimes it was a perfectly healthy pregnancy in a difficult life situation. Sometimes it was the result of sexual assault. Sometimes it was just bad timing.

"You can't judge, because you never know how you'd be in that situation. I don't believe in abortion for any reason, but I've never been in their shoes. I can't judge them. Nobody really knows what they'd do until they get there."

His words always stuck with me. And he was right. We can preach and pray all we like, but if we ever find ourselves in the position of having an unwanted pregnancy, we don't *really* know how we'd be. We hope we'd stick to our convictions no matter what the situation, but it doesn't always work out that way.

Consider these lyrics:

Mary got pregnant from a kid named Tom, said he was in love
He said, "Don't worry about a thing, baby doll, I'm the man you've been dreaming of."
But three months later he say he won't date her or return her calls
And she swear, "God damn, if I find that man I'm cutting off his balls."
Then she heads for the clinic and she gets some static walking in through the door
They call her a killer, and they call her a sinner, and they all her a whore
God forbid you ever had to walk a mile in her shoes

Cause then you really might know what it's like to have to choose[1]

Abortion is an ugly word to many people. It makes a lot of Christians uncomfortable, and rightly so if your view of personhood begins before birth. Jesus didn't say anything about abortions directly – it wasn't even an option when he walked the earth – yet it's fair to say that the Bible values life before birth. However, Jesus *did* say a lot about judgment. We are told quite clearly not to judge others in many places in the Bible.[2]

The pro-life vs pro-choice debate will rage on forever, but regardless of the outcome, let's nor forget to care for the women and men who have had their lives changed by an unwanted pregnancy. It's a hard situation, and their lives will never be the same, no matter which path is taken. It can be heartbreaking to watch a woman choose to deliberately end a pregnancy, but let's not be so arrogant to think we'd do better in her shoes. As my old preceptor said, he's seen many couples choose abortion when they were adamantly opposed to it before getting pregnant. It's sobering to consider that we never really know what we'd do till we get there.

Summary

This section was heavy. I won't offer an ethical conclusion for you. The goal here was simply to present information so you can be reasonably informed to choose on your own when personhood begins. You and your partner must discuss, pray, talk to people you trust, and decide what you're comfortable with. If you're not

---

[1] Everlast, "What it's like" (song). Warner Chappell Music Inc, Universal Music Publishing Group, 1998.

[2] Matthew 7:1-2; Luke 6:37; Romans 2:1; Romans 14:1-4, 10, 13; James 4:12

sure, that's okay. If you change your mind, that's okay too. It can be a big decision, but it doesn't have to be.

Go take a break: grab a coffee, take a walk, watch something funny. When you come back, we'll get into the real reason you're reading this book.

Let's talk about birth control.

Part 3: The Methods

Introduction

Now for the section you've been waiting for. We'll go through basics of the main methods of birth control. There are five general categories: conservative, barrier, hormonal, long term (IUD), and permanent.

When assessing how effective a particular method is, doctors cite the overall chances of getting pregnant within one year. For example, birth control pills are about 93% effective. That means of 100 sexually-active couples on birth control pills, 93 won't be pregnant at the end of the year. They fail to prevent pregnancy 7% of the time.

We'll talk about hormones again in this section, specifically estrogen and progesterone. However, the actual hormones used in birth control can be any number of synthetic estrogens or progesterones. I won't bore you with the real names of the medications. Just know that when we say "estrogen" it can refer to various medications in the estrogen family of drugs, while "progesterone" can mean any number of commercially available progesterone-like medications.

Throughout all this talk about birth control, please keep in mind that nothing you read here replaces the individualized advice of a doctor you trust.

All that being said, let's begin with the simplest method.

Conservative

Women are most fertile from Day 12-14 of their cycle, so avoiding intercourse or using barrier methods mid-cycle can reduce the chances of getting pregnant. This is called Natural Family Planning. On the other hand, the opposite approach – planned intercourse at the most fertile times – can be used to *increase* the chances of getting pregnant.

Natural Family Planning depends on the changing fertility within a woman's monthly cycle. It also depends on a single egg being released each cycle. The egg has limited opportunity to be fertilized so that it can be ready for implantation five days later. This fertilization window is about 12-24 hours after release from the ovary. Sperm lasts 3-5 days after intercourse, so timing intercourse to avoid this window of high fertility can reduce the chances of pregnancy.

To do this, you have to monitor your cycle. Your body experiences various symptoms depending on where you are in your

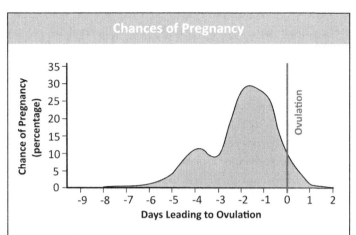

Figure 4: The chances of getting pregnant are highest in the few days leading up to ovulation, and they drop to nearly zero a day afterwards. That being said, women are theoretically able to get pregnant from intercourse on any given day in their cycle, but the odds are much lower than the peak-fertility week.

cycle. The most common symptoms to monitor are: bleeding (the start of your period), cervical mucous secretions, and increased body temperature.

Your options are as follows:

1. **Count the days**. Ovulation occurs fourteen days before the start of your next period, which would be Day 14 of a 28-day cycle, Day 16 of a 30-day cycle, etc. This assumes a consistent menstrual cycle.

2. **Monitor your secretions**. Vaginal mucous follows a pattern throughout your cycle. Starting with your period (Day 1), you'll have no secretions for 3-4 days. This is followed by scant cloudy secretions for 3-5 days. The mid-point is excessive clear, wet, stretchy secretions for 3-4 days immediately before, during, and after ovulation. This is when you're most fertile. Then there are no secretions again for 11-14 days until your cycle restarts.

3. **Check your temperature**. Your temperature is about half a degree Fahrenheit higher (0.3°C) in the second half of your cycle than the first half. The temperature begins to rise 1-2 days after ovulation and stays up for two weeks until your period starts. Because your temperature rises after ovulation, it's not a great predictor of when ovulation will happen – it just shows that it has *already* happened. After your temperature rises, your high-fertility window has passed and subsequent chances of getting pregnant are low. However, active infections (i.e. fever) can cause changes in temperature independent of the menstrual cycle, so simply catching a cold can throw off this method of monitoring.

Ultimately, how you keep track of your cycle is up to you and your partner. The best method is whichever one you're most comfortable with and can use correctly and consistently.

Natural Family Planning is best used by highly motivated women with regular menstrual cycles whose partner is supportive of this approach to birth control. They typically don't want to use more conventional forms of birth control for health reasons or personal choices. The couple must be able to avoid intercourse or use barrier methods on fertile days.

This method won't work well if your cycles are irregular or you're not interested in being militant about recording changes in your body. It also won't work well if your partner isn't completely on board.

The overall effectiveness can be as low as 75%. However, better results (up to 88%) are possibly by using temperature to monitor your cycle rather than just counting the days from your last period. Also, there's a learning curve. Unintended pregnancies occur more often in the first few months, before you've had a chance to figure out the finer points of your cycle. There are many computer or smart phone apps available to help you keep track of symptoms and intercourse days.

Advantage: your male partner will never be more involved and sensitive to your cycle. Some women appreciate this, others get annoyed with the constant questioning.

Advantage: it's inexpensive. There's no cost, except for condoms or other barriers during the fertile week.

Advantage: no pills, no extra hormones in your body, no procedures.

Advantage: no delay in fertility when you're ready to start trying for pregnancy.

One of the most common complaints with Natural Family Planning is that it's a lot of work. The hassle of carefully recording all the milestones in your cycle is inconvenient. It also removes spontaneity from your sex life, or at least forces you to use another form of birth control for unplanned intercourse. The time to have intercourse with the least chance of pregnancy is during your period, which is less than ideal for many couples.

Another major disadvantage is that it's not very effective. Although "perfect use" can have success rates near 90%, only about three-quarters of typical couples will be successful at preventing pregnancy over the course of a year.

Overall, Natural Family Planning isn't popular. Only about 3% of women worldwide use it as their primary method of birth control.

PULL OUT

Before modern medicine, *coitus interruptus* was essentially the only method of birth control. It's recorded in the Bible[1] and other ancient texts. The "Pull Out" or "Withdrawal" method is when the penis is withdrawn from the vaginal canal before ejaculation, so the semen isn't released inside.

---

[1] Genesis 38:9

The failure rate is upwards of 20% per year with typical use, but potentially as low as 4% with perfect use. Pull Out isn't particularly effective because a small amount of semen can leak out of the penis *before* ejaculation. Plus, "accidents" (failure to pull out in time) are rampant.

Advantages: no cost, no side effects, no medications, no devices, no need to plan around timing in cycle.

Disadvantage: less effective than most other methods, requires motivation and effort at every act.

Although up to 3% of couples worldwide use the Pull Out as their primary method of birth control, this is typically because social factors (such as limited finances) prohibit other more effective methods.

Barrier

All barrier methods are used around the time of intercourse to prevent sperm from entering the uterus. There are a number of female options, but only one male option.

CONDOMS

Modern sexual education efforts have focused on condom use to prevent unwanted pregnancies and reduce the spread of sexually transmitted infections. It fits over top of the penis and collects sperm in the tip, thereby preventing it from entering the vaginal canal.

Condoms aren't perfect. Typical use leads to a pregnancy rate of 13% per year. Not great odds. They fail because they're not applied correctly, they fall off during intercourse, they burst open, or they're simply not used every time.

Advantage: they're the only method of birth control that can prevent the transmission of infections. This is often not an issue with married couples, but it's a big issue for those couples not in exclusive relationships.

Advantage: cheap, readily available, easy to use.

Advantage: doesn't affect fertility when a couple wants to try to get pregnant.

Advantage: no medication to take and no side effects, unless someone's allergic to latex.

Disadvantage: sometimes couples "forget" to use them. In the heat of the moment, correctly applying a condom may not be a high priority.

Simply put, condoms work reasonably well in the short term while using another method of birth control, but long term they're a hassle.

SPERMICIDE

The active ingredient in spermicide destroys sperm, leaving them immobile and unable to bind to an egg. It can be used alone by applying it high into the vaginal canal at least 10 minutes before intercourse. It comes as a gel, cream, foam, or embedded within a sponge. Failure rate when used alone is about 20%. Spermicide commonly causes mild skin irritation to both partners.

FEMALE BARRIER METHODS

The diaphragm is a silicone dome that fits inside the vaginal canal. It's a one-size-fits-all device that is generally soft enough to be comfortable when properly inserted. A cervical cap does the same thing, but is smaller, stiffer, and comes in a variety of sizes. Both diaphragms and cervical caps are reusable for a year or more, which means they must be washed and properly stored.

All female barrier methods are designed to work with spermicide. The spermicide jelly is applied to the device before insertion, then left in for six hours after intercourse. Spermicide modestly increases their effectiveness.

As with male condoms, female barrier methods have a high failure rate, up to 20%. They require motivation to use at every encounter and take some skill to apply correctly.

Overall, female barrier methods are not a common means of birth control. They're messy and a hassle to apply every time. Combine that with their high failure rate and it's no wonder they're unpopular.

Hormones

Remember those two hormones we learned about earlier? Estrogen and progesterone. That's what hormonal birth control uses to override the menstrual cycle. You'll also remember that the trigger for ovulation is a surge of hormones from the brain. That's because the brain ultimately controls the menstrual cycle. However, when estrogen and progesterone are taken as medication, it fools the brain into giving up control of the ovaries, and the brain hormones don't surge to trigger ovulation. That's essentially how hormonal birth control works, by preventing the release of an egg from the ovaries. If there's no ovulation, there's no chance of pregnancy.

THE PILL

The most popular form of hormonal birth control is what doctors call oral contraceptives (OCP), but we'll just call The Pill. It's a tablet, containing both estrogen and progesterone, taken daily for three weeks to prevent ovulation. Then there's a "sugar pill" (without hormones) for a week to trigger menstruation – the drop off of hormones signals the time for your period to start. Packages of birth control pills have enough pills for four weeks[1] of medication, but only three weeks' worth have actual hormones. You just have to take a pill every day and the cycle will sort itself out.

As we stated, the main way birth control pills work is by preventing ovulation. That's what the estrogen does. However, the progesterone component also thickens the mucous plug in the cervix (to help block sperm from entering the uterus), and makes the uterine lining less favorable to implant an embryo, just in case ovulation occurs. Overall, birth control pills are about 93% effective. Most failures are due to not taking the pills every day, especially in the first week of the cycle.

Birth control pills can help with a number of other medical conditions besides preventing pregnancy. Acne is one of them: your skin typically improves when on hormonal birth control. Menorrhagia is another.

Menorrhagia, what a fitting term. Women who suffer from this have *raging* periods: painful cramping and heavy bleeding that causes them to miss school/work. The bleeding can be so bad that it causes anemia (low blood count). Symptoms can be debilitating. If this is you, know that there's help available. Talk to your doctor.

Historically, the dose of estrogen in birth control pills was really high, causing all sorts of nasty side effects. But over time, the dose has decreased, making The Pill much more tolerable. Side effects are usually mild and short-lived. Breast tenderness, nausea, bloating, and irregular bleeding are common but usually subside. Coming off of birth control pills can be miserable for a few months

---

[1] Most birth control pills come in cycles of 28 days. However, some formulations come as 35-day or 90-day cycles. Others still have no cycle, but provide a constant low dose of hormones so there is no period at all.

until your body gets used to cycling on its own again. However, one of the most common complaints is "I just don't like how they make me feel." Simple as that. "Moody" or "icky" or "just weird" – some women don't feel quite right on oral contraceptives. As with taking any medication, if a side effect doesn't sit well with you, get off it and find something else. But overall, birth control pills are well-tolerated by most women.

There are a number of medical reasons why your doctor may *not* prescribe The Pill. Specifically, these are conditions that can make oral contraceptives dangerous. These include:

- uncontrolled high blood pressure
- prior clots in your legs or lungs
- prior stroke or heart attack
- severe liver failure or liver cancer
- gall bladder disease
- migraines with aura
- active breast cancer
- cigarette smoking with age over 35

If you have any of these, taking estrogen may not be a good choice for you – talk to your doctor about it.

THE PATCH

Hormones can also be delivered in other ways. Instead of taking a pill by mouth every day, an adhesive patch is applied to the skin weekly for three weeks, then nothing for the fourth week. Three weeks on, one week off. The hormone-free week triggers a period in the same way that "sugar pills" do.

Because The Patch uses the same type of hormones as The Pill, their side effects are virtually the same. Additionally, The Patch can cause mild skin irritation under the adhesive.

Advantage: 96-99% effective. This improvement over birth control pills is likely due to not forgetting doses. Weekly dosing with a patch is typically easier than daily dosing with a pill. Women are instructed to pick a day of the week to be their "patch change day" – Sundays are common, so periods don't start over the weekend.

Disadvantage: patches may occasionally detach. The adhesive is quite strong – only 1 in 50 will fall off during the week. Exercise, heavy sweating, swimming, and hot tubs don't seem to affect adhesion. However, if it comes off within the first 24 hours of putting it on, it can be stuck back on where it was initially. If the patch falls off more than 24 hours after it was put on, it must be replaced with a new one, and this day of the week becomes the new patch change day.

Disadvantage: patches may be visible. It's typically applied to the buttock, abdomen, upper arms, or chest – somewhere discreet. Don't put it on your breast, since the estrogen can cause increased tenderness in nearby estrogen-sensitive breast tissue.

THE RING

Unlike patches, which must be changed weekly, a vaginal ring delivers hormone for three weeks straight. Each ring gets inserted high in the vaginal canal and stays there for 21 days, after which it's removed for a week. A new ring goes in at the start of every cycle.

It's 97% effective at preventing pregnancy during the year, with most failures related to incorrect usage.

Side effects are similar to other hormonal methods – primarily nausea and breast tenderness. It can occasionally cause vaginal irritation and increased discharge, but it's usually mild.

Advantage: no pills to take, no patch to be seen. It's invisible and relatively easy to use. Also, The Ring tends to be forgiving if it's not inserted or removed exactly on time – not like forgetting your birth control pills for a couple of days.

Disadvantage: some women aren't comfortable with an object in their vaginal canal, or with inserting/removing it.

Progesterone Injection

Unlike the hormonal methods that operate on a monthly cycle, the progesterone injection suppresses ovulation and periods altogether for as long as you're on it. Progesterone also makes mucous in the cervix thicker (more difficult for sperm to enter the uterus) and the uterine lining unfavorable for implantation. There's no estrogen, just a long-acting progesterone that gets injected every three months. It's 94% effective at preventing pregnancy.

Progesterone thins the uterine lining. This makes implantation of an embryo much less likely, if an egg somehow gets released and fertilized. However, it also makes breakthrough bleeding ("spotting") a common side effect.

Because it's an injection, you'll need to visit your doctor every three months to have it administered. For your first injection, it should be done within a week of your period starting. If you're late getting to your doctor for a repeat injection, you should use another form of birth control beyond 14 weeks. Pregnancy is unlikely up to 18 weeks after injection, but it's possible. Early repeat injection usually isn't an issue.

A big advantage of the progesterone injection is that it has no estrogen. Some women can't have estrogen for a number of reasons (see page 56). Other advantages include:

- ✓ No regular period (excellent choice for those who normally have heavy menstrual bleeding)
- ✓ No pills, no patch, no ring, and no at-home maintenance

Disadvantage: it can take a while to become fertile again. Although the progesterone injection is only supposed to last three months, it can take much longer to restore a regular cycle and ovulation. That means fertility might be delayed a year or more after your last injection.

There was some concern that bones can get brittle with years of progesterone injections, especially in teenagers whose bones are still developing. However, once the progesterone is discontinued, bone density tends to rebound back to normal. As well, the decrease in bone density is similar to what normally occurs naturally during pregnancy or breastfeeding.

Overall, progesterone injections work well if you don't want to get pregnant for at least a couple years, and you don't mind seeing the doctor every few months.

Summary

Hormonal contraception is readily accessible and relatively easy to use. However you choose to take the medication – pills, patch, ring, or injection – ovulation is prevented to reduce the chances of pregnancy considerably. Hormones are currently the most popular form of reversible birth control, but IUDs usage is quickly catching up.

Long Term

A number of devices can be implanted within the body to prevent pregnancy for years at a time. After removal, which can occur at any time, ovulation quickly resumes and you can potentially get pregnant right away. This is a big advantage over progesterone injections, which can take months – or even a year or more – to wear off.

These devices are either inserted in the uterus (IUD) or under the skin.

IUD

Intrauterine Device (IUD) is scary-sounding name, but it's a popular option for long-acting, reversible birth control. The device is a little plastic "T" that sits in the uterus for up to five years, slowly releasing low levels of either progesterone or copper into the uterus. It's just over an inch long and has two plastic strings hanging off the bottom. The strings hang just outside the cervix (not outside the vagina) for easy removal later on.

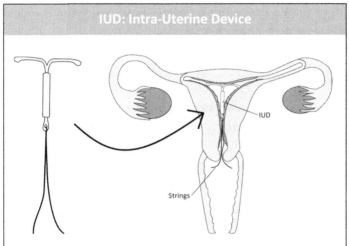

Figure 5: An IUD is a little plastic "T" that gives off medication. It's flexible and comfortable (you can't feel it) when inserted, but the insertion itself can be a challenge.

They work in two ways: the physical presence of the IUD in the uterus, plus the effect of the medication on the uterine lining. In terms of its physical presence, any device in the uterus causes a low level of inflammation, which is toxic to sperm and eggs. It also impairs implantation.

The addition of progesterone or copper also prevents pregnancy. Copper increases inflammation (just in the uterine lining, not around the body), slows down sperm, and – if all else fails – impairs implantation. There has been some concern that copper IUDs "cause abortions" every cycle, but this is highly unlikely. The general consensus is that they work primarily by preventing fertilization rather than just preventing implantation. However, to be completely honest, nobody's exactly sure how exactly copper IUDs work. They just do.[1]

Conversely, the way progesterone IUDs work is well understood. In addition to the inflammation the device causes, progesterone thickens the mucous plug in the cervix (which blocks sperm from entering the uterus) and thins the lining of the uterus to prevent implantation. By and large, neither type of IUD prevents ovulation. Instead, it disrupts the viability of sperm, eggs, and embryos.

One of the main advantages of IUDs is how effective they are. Over 99% of couples with an IUD won't get pregnant over the course of the year. That's more effective than any other non-permanent method of birth control.

Other benefits:

- ✓ No regular maintenance, no pills, no regular doctor visits
- ✓ Long-lasting: the same device prevents pregnancy for five years or more

In terms of cost, IUDs can be pricey, especially progesterone. However, the overall cost of an IUD is less expensive than The Pill; they pay for themselves after two years of not buying hormonal birth control.

The biggest downside of IUDs is the insertion. It involves a speculum exam, like a pap smear, but the instruments go further.

---

[1] The lack of a definitive explanation on how a medical intervention works can be unnerving. But to put it in perspective, the same issue exists with the medication acetaminophen (also called paracetamol, or Tylenol). It relieves fever and mild pain, likely through inhibiting inflammation in the body, but nobody's really sure how. It just works. And it's one of the most commonly used medications worldwide. Chances are you've taken it yourself.

A doctor dilates the cervix (painful) and inserts the applicator (a plastic tube, about the diameter of a drinking straw). The IUD is positioned in the uterus and the applicator comes out. There's usually bleeding for a day or two, which can vary from light spotting to a heavy period. Serious complications are uncommon. The whole procedure by an experienced doctor takes less than a few minutes. If you've ever delivered a baby vaginally, the insertion is usually less painful.

Sometimes IUDs fall out, often within the first month. This happens in up to 6% of cases. Occasionally IUDs don't align themselves correctly in the uterus, that is, they become mispositioned. This happens in about 10% of cases, causing pain and irregular bleeding. If this happens, the IUD needs to come out. It's a hassle. Whether an IUD falls out on its own or gets removed by a doctor, it's no longer sterile and needs to be replaced.

Whenever a couple wants to start trying for pregnancy, a doctor performs another speculum exam and pulls the IUD out (relatively pain-free). After that, the couple is good to go. The birth control is rapidly reversible. However, sometimes the strings retract into the uterus and minor surgery is needed to fish it out.

That being said, if a woman manages to get pregnant with an IUD in place, it may cause problems during the pregnancy. If it's early in the pregnancy, your doctor may opt to pull the IUD out, but it can also be left in place if the risks of removal outweigh the benefits. It's not the end of the world get pregnant with an IUD in the uterus – many obstetricians will deliver a healthy baby with an IUD embedded in its placenta sometime in their career.

In terms of side effects, bleeding and cramping are most common, especially in the first few months. Most women feel fine by six months. Sometimes the plastic strings can cause problems. They hang just outside the cervix and can feel pokey. If they're too long, they can poke into the vaginal wall, in which case they can be trimmed shorter. If they're too short, the penis can get poked during intercourse – not fun for your partner. To fix this, a doctor can try to push the strings aside or they can be cut flush with the cervix.

Progesterone IUDs come in various doses. The most common one lasts five years, but lower dose IUDs may only be good for three years. In addition to birth control, progesterone IUDs improve painful, crampy periods. Many women find their periods get lighter, shorter, and less crampy with a progesterone IUD in place. Sometimes your period can disappear altogether for six months or more. Intermittent spotting is common but rarely dangerous.

Copper IUDs are the same size and shape as progesterone IUDs. Unless you have an allergy to copper (rare), any female with a healthy uterus can get one. They tend to be less expensive, but not many doctors recommend them because they usually make periods heavier and crampier. This often improves over the first six months, but if heavy periods are already a problem for you, a copper IUD may not be a good choice.

Overall, if you can get past the miserable insertion, IUDs are well-tolerated, low maintenance, and highly effective.

Progesterone Implant

Instead of a device within your uterus, a small plastic rod can be implanted under the skin, which slowly releases progesterone and prevents ovulation. It's about the size and shape of a matchstick, but flexible. It usually gets placed just under the skin on the inside of the upper arm.

The insertion procedure is considerably less invasive than that of an IUD. A doctor numbs the area with freezing (local anesthetic), then the introducer pierces the skin and is gently burrowed under the surface. Once in all the way, the introducer is withdrawn, leaving the implant behind. The small hole is bandaged; no stitches needed. The whole procedure takes a few minutes and leaves a tiny scar when healed.

Like IUDs, progesterone implants can be removed at any time. After your doctor makes a small incision, the implant is pulled out from under the skin. Again, no stitches needed, just a small bandage. Periods get lighter or disappear altogether.

Progesterone implants are supposed to be replaced every three years, but they may be effective for longer.

The main disadvantage is their cost – considerably more than other methods. Also, because they're relatively new, your doctor may not be familiar with it.

Permanent

There a number of procedures that can sterilize one of the partners in a relationship. Some are done in a clinic in a matter of minutes, others require major surgery. In general, permanent methods of birth control (i.e. sterilization) are highly effective, with a failure rate well below 1%.

For men, a vasectomy cuts the tube that supplies sperm from the testicles to the urethra (*vas deferens*). However, a vasectomy isn't considered effective right away, since there can still be sperm elsewhere in the reproductive tract. A back-up method should be used until a semen analysis confirms you're "shooting blanks."

Over 90% of semen volume comes from glands in the male reproductive tract that are not disconnected by a vasectomy. After the procedure, semen will have no sperm and a slightly lower volume, but otherwise semen will be unchanged.

The procedure itself is typically performed in a clinic. The doctor injects freezing to numb the area then makes a small incision to get at the vas deferens. After the tube is cut and the ends sealed shut, the incision is closed with bandages or stitches. Serious complications are rare.

For women, a tubal ligation cuts the fallopian tube, which blocks an egg from reaching the uterus (and from sperm reaching the ovaries). This can be done with a "keyhole" surgery[1] or during a C-section. Clips are applied around the fallopian tube to block it, or a section of it is simply removed with both ends tied off.

Vasectomy and tubal ligation are both reasonably safe procedures. However, because a vasectomy can be done in a clinic without needing to put the man to sleep, it's considered the safest surgical sterilization procedure.

These procedures are considered permanent, so if there's any doubt you want to have more kids, surgical contraception isn't a good choice for you. In some cases, they can be reversed with another surgery, but this is often unsuccessful to restore fertility. Also, the reverse procedure usually isn't covered by health care plans and can be very expensive.

As with any surgery, complications include bleeding, infection, damage to surrounding structures, and chronic pain. However, long term problems are rare.

Sterilization is the most common method of birth control worldwide, second only to The Pill.

Hysterectomy

The only 100% effective surgical method of birth control is removal of the uterus (hysterectomy). Without a uterus, the vaginal canal is essentially a dead end – it's still functional for

---

[1] Laparoscopy ("keyhole" surgery) is when a few small incisions are made in the abdomen, which is then inflated. The whole surgery is performed with a camera and tools inserted through the keyholes. The recovery is faster and easier than a laparotomy (making a larger "old-school" incision).

intercourse, but there will be no periods and nowhere to for sperm to go.

Hysterectomy is never reversible. The only way to have a baby without a uterus is in vitro fertilization with a surrogate mother.[1]

Hysterectomy is a major surgery with significant associated risks. It's generally not used just to prevent pregnancy, but rather to treat various gynecological conditions.

Breastfeeding

Most new moms don't want to get pregnant right away. Breastfeeding itself can be a form of birth control for the first six months, since the hormone that stimulates milk production (prolactin) also inhibits the monthly cycle. However, this method is notoriously unreliable. After having a baby, your period should come back 3-9 months later, but keep in mind that you'll already have been fertile for two weeks before your first period. So don't rely on not having a period to reassure you that you're not yet ovulating.

Options are limited when you've got a baby to feed, since estrogen can interfere with milk production. Progesterone, however, does not.

The Mini-Pill is a birth control pill that only contains progesterone. The biggest drawback is that it must be taken at the same time every day to be effective. If you're late with a dose, even by a few hours, your chances of getting pregnant go way up. Thus, it doesn't work very well for mothers of new babies, who have completely mixed up sleep-wake cycles and erratic daily

---

[1] See Part 4 on Reproductive Technology.

schedules, not to mention forgetfulness from being sleep-deprived.

If a strict pill schedule doesn't work, progesterone injections can potentially start as soon as the baby is out. There are no pills to remember, just a visit to the doctor every three months. Because it's just progesterone, there are no issues with milk supply.

Another option is an IUD. Both progesterone and copper IUDs can potentially be inserted into the uterus as early as minutes after delivery of a baby. However, because the cervix has just dilated enough to deliver a baby, IUDs get mispositioned or fall out more often if inserted immediately afterward. Alternatively, they can be put in anytime in the following weeks/months after delivery. IUDs don't interfere with breastfeeding and don't require you to remember to take pills daily, which is a big benefit for new mothers.

Finally, permanent methods are always possible. The man can get "The Snip" or the woman can get her tubes tied. Many women will have their obstetrician tie their tubes at the same time as a C-section, if they're completely done with getting pregnant.

Emergency Contraception

Accidents happen. In the case of intercourse without any birth control on board, there are a few options to a prevent pregnancy from occurring. To be clear, emergency contraception doesn't cause an abortion of an existing pregnancy. All of these methods work by preventing ovulation, fertilization, or implantation.

The Morning-After Pill, also called Plan B, is one or two doses of hormones taken after unprotected intercourse to prevent pregnancy. The most common Morning-After Pills are progesterone alone, but an estrogen-progesterone combination also works. You need to take it within three days of the event, but the sooner the better. If taken before ovulation, progesterone can prevent the release of an egg from the ovary. If you'll remember, a hormone surge from the brain triggers ovulation, but progesterone can prevent this surge and thereby prevent ovulation. No egg released means no pregnancy. However, this only works if taken earlier than the day of ovulation. Once the brain hormones surge, an egg is likely to be released whether you take progesterone or not.

If an egg is already released or fertilized, hormones won't interfere with implantation. Nor will hormones interfere with an embryo that has already implanted.

Side effects of progesterone-only pills are generally mild: headache, abdominal pain, nausea, or menstrual cycle irregularity. However, the side effects of the combined estrogen-progesterone pills are awful: nausea and vomiting are common. Most women who get prescribed the combination pill should get a prescription for an anti-nauseant as well.

Overall, the Morning-After Pill works most of the time, with a failure rate of about 2%.

Copper IUDs, however, when inserted within five days of unprotected sex, prevent over 99% of pregnancies. The copper IUD for emergency contraception gets recommended by doctors more than the Morning-After Pill, mostly because it can be left in place to provide ongoing birth control. Most women who have it inserted after an "oops" are happy with it later on down the road.

In general, your only two methods of emergency contraception are The Morning After Pill and a copper IUD. Either way, the sooner it's used, the more likely it'll work.

Abstinence

After all this talk about birth control, it's worth mentioning here that abstinence is the only sure-fire, 100% effective way to prevent pregnancy. Short of a miracle,[1] if you don't have sex, you won't get pregnant.[2]

If you're reading this book, you've likely crossed abstinence off your list already, but it's always worth considering. Apart from a hysterectomy, nothing else is as effective.

Summary

As far as we can tell, none of the forms of birth control cause an abortion. That is, none of these methods end an established (successfully implanted) pregnancy. They all primarily work by preventing fertilization, the union of sperm and egg. The only exception is perhaps the copper IUD, which *likely* prevents fertilization, but we can't be certain.

In terms of popularity, The Pill is the most widely used method of reversible birth control, but IUD usage has been steadily increasing for years. Many couples use a variety of methods over the course of their relationship, depending on the season of life they're in. Talk to each other, talk to God, and talk to your doctor. In medicine, there's always an aspect of trial-and-error to find a therapy that fits each person. Sometimes the only way to discover what works (or *doesn't* work) is to give it a shot.

---

[1] Pregnancy without intercourse has only occurred once in the history of the world, and it was under quite unique circumstances. See Matthew 1:18.

[2] This is assuming there's no reproductive technology (artificial insemination, *in vitro* fertilization, etc.).

Whatever your goals for birth control, there's a method that's right for you and your partner. As we said earlier, your choice should be well-understood, easy to use, and (most of all) keep your conscience clear.

Part 4: Reproduction Technology

Introduction

This is a bonus section. I hope you and your partner never need to know this, but the harsh reality is that some couples have great difficulty getting pregnant or carrying a baby to term. It can be a difficult journey, but reproductive technology may be the only option for a couple to conceive and deliver a healthy baby. It's expensive, somewhat risky, and fraught with challenges. It's also an emotional rollercoaster.

As I said, I hope you never need to travel down this road.

Options

When we talk about reproductive technology, we mean any artificial assistance with getting pregnant. It's includes any procedure that handles sperm and eggs outside the body. There are two main reasons why reproductive technology is used: inability to get pregnant by conventional means (i.e. intercourse) and high risk of genetic abnormalities.

In most cases, fertilization occurs in a lab, not inside the woman's reproductive tract. However, implantation of the developing embryo must still occur in a healthy uterus for a pregnancy to be successful. After that, it's up to the uterus and growing fetus to make it to term.

We'll be brief in our discussion here, since the technology is always advancing and can be quite complicated. The invasiveness is highly variable, depending on the problem with conception that the couple is trying to overcome. We'll start our discussion with the least invasive.

Artificial Insemination, AI

Instead of intercourse putting sperm into the woman, artificial insemination puts it there with a syringe. The sperm is typically from a donor, used to overcome male infertility (abnormal or absent sperm). The donor sperm is injected into the vaginal canal (essentially the same result as intercourse) or directly into the uterus.

In Vitro Fertilization, IVF

In vivo is Latin for "in the living." *In vitro* means "in glass." During *in vitro* fertilization, the sperm and egg are combined in a lab. For this to happens, sperm and eggs must first be collected from the parents.

Sperm collection is usually easy. But in the case of a man's inability to produce enough healthy sperm, the sperm he does have can be pulled out directly from the testicle with a needle (a doctor will do this).

Egg retrieval is more complicated. The woman goes on hormonal medications to stimulate the ovaries to produce many eggs in a single cycle, not just one. Then, under the guidance of an ultrasound, a doctor will insert a needle into the ovaries and suck out the contents of each follicle, each of which should produce a viable egg.

As we discussed, fertilization occurs outside the female reproductive tract. Sometimes this is as simple as putting the sperm and egg together in the same container. If this doesn't work, a sperm can be injected directly into an egg.

After the sperm and egg combine, the embryo is allowed to grow for nearly a week before being transferred into a uterus. Many embryos are prepared in the lab, but only one or two are inserted into the uterus in any given cycle. Leading up to embryo transfer, the woman goes on hormones again to make her uterine lining as ready for pregnancy as possible. In the case of a woman with abnormalities in her uterus, a surrogate uterus may be used.

Ideally, the embryo implants in the uterine lining and a pregnancy occurs. However, after all that trouble, not all injected embryos successfully implant. IVF failure is common.

In vitro fertilization can help a couple overcome a number of barriers to fertility, such as abnormal sperm, problems with the fallopian tubes, and early menopause.

CRYOPRESERVATION

This brings us to the issue of what to do with unused or unwanted products. Not all sperm and eggs used in reproductive technology get used. Similarly, not all embryos created in the lab get used either. A couple my become pregnant on their first attempt at IVF, or limited finances may prevent further attempts. As well, couples may want to save their embryos for a future date when they're ready for another pregnancy, or perhaps donate them to other couples who cannot produce viable embryos on their own. Whatever the reason, labs often have extra "reproductive material" they need to store for prolonged periods.

It all gets frozen.

In general, freezing these cells – whether eggs, sperm, or embryos – doesn't increase birth defects or developmental abnormalities. They can be thawed and used without major issue at a later date.

However, ethics come into play when nobody wants the embryos anymore. If a couple's beliefs dictate that personhood begins at fertilization, the prospect of discarding unused embryos can be upsetting. Likewise for donating them for research. For this reason, it's important that every couple go into the process of IVF with a clear understanding what will happen with their unused embryos.

CLONING

There are a lot of movies about cloning, where a person is made from the genetic material of a single parent. In 1996, a sheep named Dolly made history as the first successful clone of a large mammal. She had three mothers: one provided the egg, another the DNA, and a third carried the cloned embryo in her uterus.

Cloning works like this: an egg has its nucleus (with the half-set of DNA from the mother) removed, then a new nucleus from the parent cell is inserted. The parent nucleus is from neither an egg nor a sperm, but has a *full* set of DNA, identical to that of the single parent. The egg, now with all the genetic material it needs, starts replicating and forms an embryo. It gets transferred into a uterus and after the pregnancy is complete, a clone is born.

Cloning is terribly inefficient and has many challenges. Dolly was the only successful lamb that survived to adulthood in 277 attempts. Granted, technology has advanced considerably since then, but the whole process is still tedious and risky.

Since Dolly, many other mammals have been cloned, including monkeys, which are genetically similar to humans. However, as far as we know, a human has not yet been cloned.

Dolly's birth also opened the door for stem cell research, which is when cells are produced that have the ability to grow into any type of tissue. That's essentially what embryos are – undifferentiated "anything" cells. Stem cell technology can potentially cure type 1 diabetes. Future development may allow for the treatment of heart disease, blindness, dementia, and cancer.

Genetic Screening

Some couples are at high risk of producing children with genetic defects. Before implantation, embryos can be tested and selected for transfer based on their genetic profile. Unwanted embryos, with undesirable genetic profiles, are discarded.

The ethics here can get murky here. Pre-implantation genetic screening opens up the possibility of having a "savior sibling." If an existing child requires a bone marrow or organ donor, the parents can potentially select an embryo with a compatible genetic profile. After birth, this new child may have the means to save their diseased older sibling. There's also the potential to select genetic traits unrelated to disease, such as gender and eye color. This leads to the prospect of "designer babies." On the other hand, embryos can also be selected that *have* a disability, such as parents with dwarfism who intentionally want a child with the same condition. Furthermore, DNA within an embryo can be edited to modify its genetic makeup in virtually any way. This is generally prohibited by law, as gene editing may have unintentional consequences later on in development.

As you can see, genetic screening opens up a whole can of worms that many people, both in science and religion, are uncomfortable with. But is it morally wrong? Hard to say.

Summary

Infertility is a heart-wrenching struggle for many couples. Many women (and their husbands) in the Bible suffered from infertility, including Sarah, Rebekah, Hannah, and Elizabeth. Rachel, the wife of Jacob, felt like she would die if she continued to suffer from barrenness.[1]

Her agony is not unique.

Advice on reproductive technology is beyond the scope of this book. Many couples have been able to parent their own biologic children because of these advanced procedures, when a generation ago it would have been impossible. It's far from a sure bet, but reproductive technology can at least provide an option to overcome infertility. Indeed, most couples who struggle with infertility will try just about anything to have children of their own.

---

[1] Genesis 30:1

Conclusion

Final Words

That's it! We're finally at the end. Contraception, and the science and ethics that surround it, can be an overwhelming topic. Flying through the basics, like we did here, can feel like drinking from a firehose. If you've managed to read this far, good for you. Hopefully you've found all this helpful in making an informed decision about birth control.

At the risk of repeating myself yet again, talk to your doctor about your goals and priorities for birth control. The personalized advice of your doctor is irreplaceable and should be your ultimate source of information. If anything they say contradicts something you've read in these pages, go with your doctor over this book.

Medicine is constantly evolving. The information here is meant to be a guide on the basics of reproduction, ethics, birth control, and reproduction technology. It's not a definitive medical resource or a code of ethics. Also, *Birth Control For Christians* isn't meant to decide anything for you, rather it's simply here to inform you. If nothing else, this book would be an awkward (yet helpful) gift for someone who's about to get married.

An in-law perhaps?

Also, we've already touched on this briefly, but the personal decisions of others aren't something we should judge. Opinions on the ethics surrounding reproduction can be volatile. Discuss this with whoever you like, but be careful: you might be surprised at how easily close friends and family will be offended (or become offensive) regarding different points of view.

However, let's end on a positive note. The reason to use birth control, after all, is to enjoy a positive experience without having to plan for a subsequent pregnancy. The Bible says this:

"How beautiful is your love, my sister, my bride…
Your lips, my bride, drip honey; honey and milk are under your tongue."[1]

"I am my beloved's, and his desire is for me.
Come, my beloved, let's go out to the fields…
There I'll give you my love."[2]

God made sex a good thing. If birth control helps you enjoy it within a loving, committed relationship, then by all means use it. Make an informed decision with your partner on whatever method seems best. Then hop in bed with the one you love with a clear conscience.

Enjoy!

---

[1] Song of Songs 4:10-11
[2] Song of Songs 7:10-12

Also by DB Ryen

BIBLES:

The Story of Jesus: All Four Gospels In One (Study Bible)
The Story of Jesus: All Four Gospels In One (Just The Word)

HISTORICAL (BIBLICAL) FICTION:

Never The Same: Twelve Lives Changed By Jesus

CHILDREN'S STORIES:

Rory the Knight and the Giant Squid

Rory the Knight and the Anaconda

Rory the Knight and the Grumpy Old Alligator

Spaceman Bren and the Slime Monster

Spaceman Bren and the Planet of Apes

Download samples and more at www.dbryen.com

> *I made the journey of a lifetime to carry the cross for a criminal, not knowing that it was he who was actually carrying it for me.*
> — Simon of Cyrene

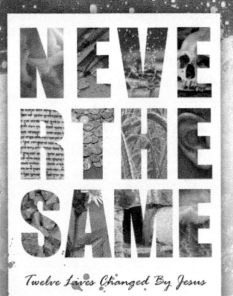

Elizabeth Peter
Jairus Lazarus
Barabbas
Lesion Simon
Talya Joseph
Levi
Azriel Malchus

www.dbryen.com

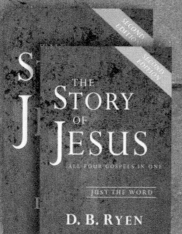

Made in the USA
Middletown, DE
23 October 2021